Spirituality and Women's Health

A definitive guide to living intentionally, healthy and strong

Copyright © 2019

Table of Contents

Introduction

Every woman is born special!

The statement above isn't meant to induce butterflies in your stomach alone because it is a fact. From birth, a woman starts to exhibit unique and distinctive traits, but the older she gets, the more exposed she is to the world.

Now exposure brings a lot into a woman's life while empowering her to deal with the real world; it also exposes her to a lot of issues that could lead to health challenges if not properly managed. As women, we often wonder if we can ever return to the state we were before this "Exposure."

The truth is we can always go back to that state, but it requires dedication, commitment, and intentionality long-term. Being a healthy and wholesome woman involves a lot of work that cuts across fitness, relationships, spirituality, etc.

Every woman needs to strike a balance between varying aspects of her life to be truly healthy. By healthy, we are not solely referring to the body but the entire makeup of the woman. We are considering physical, mental, emotional, and spiritual health.

A lot of times, the world teaches women to consider their physical health as paramount and disregard other aspects. While physical fitness is essential, there is a need to develop yourself into a TOTAL WOMAN who is entirely healthy.

For example, would you say a woman who struggles with depression is healthy? Of course, no! Now depression is not a matter of physical health, it is within the realms of mental health, but if we don't address such issues, we cannot say a person is completely healthy.

While some women have it high in an area, they may struggle with another region. This book aims to help every woman strike a balance between all aspects of women's health. This book contains the most detailed and well-researched ideas that will give you the much-needed boost you require.

In this material, you will also discover a chapter on spirituality, which is a very vital aspect of health and wellness; some persons don't take seriously. Spirituality is at the core of everything we do as women, and it contributes immensely to the women's health narrative.

What you have with this book is a combined package of everything you need to turn your life around for good. It is not enough for us to exist; as women, we've got to THRIVE and BLOOM like butterflies. For that to happen, we must understand the right kind of information and use it deliberately.

Are you ready to get started on the journey towards better and long-lasting health in all areas? We will begin with a generalized concept in chapter one and build up to other areas. Enjoy the read!

Chapter One
The general concept of women's health

Our journey begins with a broad yet different approach to the idea of women's health. What does it mean when we say a woman is healthy? Are we referring to her mental state? Physical condition? There are varying aspects.

But the idea we want you to grasp here is that good health means completeness. Good health refers to the concept of a woman being whole with every area, and for any woman to achieve this level of wholeness, she must take action.

Women's health is an idea that speaks of the possibility of having it all even beyond medicine or physical health. It relates to being happy, whole, and excited about life all at the same time.

There are women with a clean bill of health from their doctors who are not living authentic lives because they lack certain other aspects while some others are happy but have a severe health challenge.

The general concept of women's health speaks of the woman with good physical and mental health. In the world today, it has been made to seem like women can't have both because life throws curveballs. But you must believe that if you stick to the right principles long-term, you can have it all.

Women's health also refers to the concept of being intentional about life because you are aware that your actions and inactions have repercussions. This notion plays out like this; being conscious of health will propel you to make good choices; such significant decisions will have an impact on your general health.

So we want you to know that after reading this book, your thought process about health will be completely different from the norm. It isn't solely about terminal diseases or headaches but also about how you feel internally and how you relate to the world.

This realization will cause you to always check on yourself based on these criteria to know if you are truly healthy. There is also the spiritual side of things that teaches you the religious implications of specific actions on your health.

So what are the essential areas to consider when talking about women's health?

1. Mental health

Mental health is the state of your well-being mentally and how you relate with yourself. Recently the world has focused a lot on mental health because people silently deal with adverse mental health challenges such as depression.

A woman struggling with her mental health will ultimately become physically ill because there is a connection between the psychological and physical aspects of our lives.

2. Psychological health

Psychological health is a combination of emotional, behavioral, and social well-being of a person. This aspect deals with the ability to function effectively in society through positively inspired behavior.

The state of your psychological health can be affected by the people you relate with, those you meet, and how you react to events happening around you. For a woman to attain excellent psychological health, she must be intentional about it and monitor her thought process as well.

3. Physical health

Physical health relates to your body and how healthy it is generally. Excellent physical fitness is the absence of illness and the availability of a robust immune system. When a woman has excellent physical health, it means she is in the right place with her body and doesn't need to rely on medication long-term.

4. Emotional health

Emotional health is NOT the same as mental health, even though both terms are used interchangeably. Emotional health is all about our emotions and how to attune to our feelings. Good psychological health will help a woman become resilient, self-aware, authentic, and content.

The attributes mentioned above helps a woman achieve balance with her health and total wellness. Please note that having excellent emotional health doesn't mean you will be happy all the time or that you are free from negative emotions. It means that you are highly aware of your emotional state enough to ascertain when things are not right and dealing with it effectively.

5. Spiritual health

Spiritual health and its connection to diseases will be discussed in detail in the last chapter of this book. But first, you should know that there are religious implications connected to your feelings.

We don't address spiritual health a lot because it is a sensitive area, but it is also crucial. When you read through the last chapter, you will understand why it is so important.

Every concept mentioned above will be discussed in varying ways in the chapters below because the goal is for you to achieve perfect health.

This chapter is a foundational one that provided fundamental insight into the direction of the book. You will read about physical health for sure, but the content wouldn't be restricted to that alone. You will also find other valuable aspects that, when put together, creates a ripple effect for positive manifestations in your life.

The next section takes a more direct aim at an aspect of women's health that is very crucial for all women. While this aspect can be disturbing for some women, we believe that it is an opportunity to live your best life in a significant way.

Chapter Two
How to stay healthy while aging gracefully

A significant concern for most women relates to aging because we all want to look great even though time doesn't wait for us. Aside from still wanting to show up with a great bikini body, we want to be healthy internally, as well. Before talking about the main content of this chapter, let's crush an erroneous idea.

The wrong idea is that women should become afraid to age because aging is associated with a lot of negative changes. Well, this approach isn't entirely accurate! Some women age gracefully, they get into their 40's, 50's, and 60' with so much strength and beauty, thus smashing the idea that aging is problematic.

If you do the right things you are supposed to do, you wouldn't be worried about aging. On the contrary, you will be excited about every birthday because you are loving life. Now you should know that when aging, your life has to come full circle in every sense of the word.

Coming full circle means all aspects of your life are in sync such that you are radiant with joy. Aging comes with its unique challenges, but if you know what to do at this time of your life, the problems will be a walk in the park.

Getting older doesn't mean you will have a series of medical issues, poor quality of life, and sad days. Yes, aging brings changes, but you can become familiar with the changes that happen in your body while maintaining good health.

The remaining part of this chapter will focus on some essential steps and ideas you can implement to age gracefully. Some of the ideas you will discover below are not new concepts, but there are powerful when put to use intentionally.

How women can age gracefully

1. Limit alcoholic consumption

Alcoholic consumption has to be limited; your body's immune system is not as secure as it was when you were younger. At this age, you must consider what is most beneficial for your body and not want you "Want" to do.

2. Cut down on smoking

Smoking affects the lungs and can negatively affect your health, so now is an excellent time to put a stop to it.

3. Eat a well-balanced diet

We will discuss extensively on the importance of food to the narrative in another chapter. But before we get to that chapter, you should know that eating a well-balanced diet at this stage of your life is beyond crucial. Stop eating junk food and stick with foods that are rich in fiber, also drink a lot of water with fruits and veggies.

4. Stay socially active

To age gracefully, you cannot be isolated hence the reason for social relevance. You've got to stay engaged with friends, family, and your community by reaching out to them and attending events.

If you stay away from people, you will be closed in and miss out on a lot of meaningful events. If you've got grandkids, spend time with them, and stay connected with those you love. Make new friends, strengthen old friendships, and hold on to your network.

5. Don't neglect yourself

When we grow older, we give attention to everyone else, the kids, spouses, partners, businesses, etc. In some cases, this attention given to others makes it easier for us to neglect ourselves. But this must change if you will age gracefully, you need to strike a balance between attention on yourself and others.

Spend time with yourself, go shopping, and get that beautiful dress you've always wanted. Live fully; take care of yourself while looking out for others. Also, go for regular check-ups with your doctor, optometrist and dentists, don't neglect your health. The keyword here   is   BALANCE!

6. Listen to your body

As we grow older, a lot of things compete for our attention, and it makes it easier for us to pay less attention to our bodies. So I am urging you at this point to pay attention to your body because it is always speaking.

Don't trivialize symptoms, and if you feel a certain way, alert your doctor. Reaching your doctor doesn't mean you should always go into panic mode but pay attention to your body and observe changes.

7. Love yourself

Above all, you must love yourself because self-love is critical. Regardless of how much others like you, if you don't love yourself, you would age miserably. Love your body, your mind, values, skin, and everything that makes you unique.

Don't fall out of love with yourself because your skin looks different, or you've got some grey hair. When you look in the mirror, see the child in you, and stay in that mental state always.

Every day should be an opportunity for you to find something unique about yourself that you appreciate. When you practice self-love, you will age gracefully and beautifully.

Aging is a concept of the mind!

Yes, you are growing older, but if you feel younger in your mind, it will ultimately show forth in everything you do. Don't neglect yourself while taking care of other people, tend to your mental health, and enjoy each day as it comes.

A major determinant of good health for women long-term is exercise; in fact, we cannot complete this journey without considering the activity. The next chapter will take you through the exercise process in the most detailed way, get your fitness outfits ready!

Chapter Three
Exercise is the new oxygen!

With this book, we seek to give you a complete experience and an idea of who a healthy woman is and what you can do to achieve it. We have been discussing in general terms with the first two chapters, and from this chapter, we will be much more specific.

What better way to commence the introduction of peculiar sections if not through a chapter on exercise? Exercise is a physical activity that helps keep the body fit and healthy. We are talking about how to help women build a healthier life, and training is crucial to the discourse.

Some women get interested in exercises when they want to lose weight and stop being consistent afterward. In fact, due to the influx of so many social media opinion pieces and other fitness trends, exercise is portrayed as activities women should indulge in when seeking better weight.

But we want you to know that the assertion above isn't true! Exercise is the new oxygen because it goes beyond the weight discourse. Yes, one can lose weight through regular exercise, but training should be a part of your lifestyle with or without a desire for weight loss.

An inactive woman cannot be healthy; she might look alright on the outside but will surely have a weaker immune system. Such women are also susceptible to illnesses and diseases because they are not active. If you are keen on exercise, you will agree that it is indeed the most refreshing activity, so why wouldn't women engage in practice?

There are numerous aspects to our discussion, but listen to this, everything we will discuss connects to being fit and healthy. For example, in chapter 2, we touched upon the concept of aging gracefully. However, you cannot gracefully age if you are not fit!

As we move on to other chapters, you will find some mental, psychological, and spiritual facets of the discussion, which will be enabled when you are fit. So exercise should be taken seriously, it should be a part of your routine and something you enjoy.

In the world of exercise of fitness, there are several activities you can indulge in from taking long walks to cardio, weight lifting, hiking, etc. all of these are great, but you must do what works best for you.

Some women only feel like they will make progress with exercise when they are at the gym. But there are working mums with kids, and their responsibility to family makes it difficult for them to go to the gym. If this is your peculiar case, I would advise that you find other ways to exercise that don't conflict with your commitment to the kids.

You could use the stairs, jog around the neighborhood, take a short walk while the kids are resting, etc. the idea for you shouldn't always be to do what you "Think" will work but to do what you "Can" given the circumstance.

However, if you don't have family or wok constraints, you should challenge yourself and your body through exercise. Exercise for women is more fun when there is a variety of activities to switch from that best fits some parts of the body.

There are various technical types of exercises for women out there, and we wouldn't be able to list them all here. What you will find below is a list of some exercise routines you can do anywhere (home or in the gym) and anytime. The idea of exercise as the new oxygen takes away the previously held narrative that a person must be in a fitness group to get the benefits of exercise routines.

Fitness groups are practical (they motivate you), but we don't want to make women feel pressured. So if you feel anxious about joining a group, start at home and build your body confidence until you can join one. There is so much you can achieve at home, BUT don't stay home for too long as you may want to use some specialized gym equipment for specific exercise purposes.

Now back to the list we talked about earlier:

1. Dancing

Dancing is one of the most comfortable routines you can do anywhere, dance while cooking, dance at parties, and dance everywhere else. With simple dance steps, you can keep your body active, and if you want it to be more fun, join a dance class.

2. Jogging

Going for a jog is also a good idea, especially within your neighborhood. If you are a busy woman with a family and career commitment, you can jog early in the morning and evenings to stay fit.

3. Walking

Walking can be done at any time in the day and in more straightforward ways too. Use the stairs and avoid the elevator, park the car, and walk a distance back home, etc.

4. Running

If you've got a park nearby your home, you can use it for your morning or evening runs; you can also get a treadmill in your home that will encourage you to run in the house and do more lapses.

5. Sit-ups

Sit-ups are great if you want to lose tummy fat and increase your flexibility. Sit-ups can be done at home multiple times to tone the ab area and improve posture.

6. Weight lifting

Now for weight lifting, you can start with dumbbells at home and slowly build your stamina to take on heavier weights. When you are confident and set for a new challenge, then you may have to register at a gym for heavier loads.

7. Pushups

Pushups are great for building upper body strength, and they are a fast way to get activity done in a day. Pushups are also quick and easy to get used to the long-term. There are other higher variations of pushups, primarily if you work with a personal trainer.

Please note that the list above concentrates on elementary forms of exercise, especially for those who don't have a proper workout routine. These activities will get you geared up to take on more challenging events in the future.

To stay in shape and in excellent form, you must exercise regularly. If you've got a challenge with your weight, determine your goal wright goal, and work towards achieving it. A healthy woman is one who is also body confident and comfortable in her skin. Such a woman shows up to a meeting, strutting like the hallway is her runway, and she is ready to conquer the world because she is fit and healthy.

Besides her excellent exercise routine, the superwoman is also conscious of what she eats because she recognizes that food plays a crucial role.

The next chapter will instruct you on the basic idea of food and the role it plays in helping you maintain good health.

Chapter Four
The role of food

A balanced diet is crucial for excellent health, and women should enjoy a variety of healthy foods from all the food groups. When we are younger, it might be easier for us to get away with a lot of bad food habits, but as we grow older, we must be careful with what we eat.

At each stage of a woman's life, there are specific nutritional needs that change with time. The goal should be to know what applies to them to a particular time and stick to it.

But generally, good food is a compulsory aspect of health and wellness. How you look outwardly is a reflection of what you eat. Regardless of the artificial skin care routine, you invest in, if you are not getting the right nutrients and minerals into your body, you wouldn't have great skin.

In addition to great skin, eating right also enables you to maintain a healthy weight. Women who suffer from weight-related challenges such as obesity have been eating the wrong foods for a long time. Yes, exercise is excellent, but training with the wrong type of food will not help you.

Nutrient-dense meals provide energy for women, especially those with hectic lives. Such foods also reduce the risks of diseases while giving the immune system a significant boost. The importance of a healthy diet has led to the formation of various dietary plans today to help women eat the right foods.

Regardless of the dietary plan you decide on, you must know the required foods to eat on the program. More so, you should always speak with your doctor before adopting any plan so you can forever remain on the right eating path.

Dietary plan or not, there are some essential foods every woman should eat because of the minerals they offer the body. This type of food is known as "Superfood," and when included in meals, they boost the health of a woman.

The list of superfoods is an exhaustive one that contains a lot of vegetables, grains, fruits, etc. as such, we may not be able to mention all the foods in this chapter. But we will focus on the essential ones you can purchase wherever you are in the world.

Top ten superfoods for a healthy body

1. Quinoa

Quinoa tastes like couscous, and they contain all nine essential amino acids. This superfood keeps our muscles and organs healthy, preventing them from breaking down. Quinoa is a whole carbohydrate loaded with minerals, vitamins, and magnesium; you can find quinoa in the rice aisle when grocery shopping.

2. Kale

Kale belongs to the leafy green family that has a lot of health benefits for women. Kale is beneficial for the heart, high for the complexion, and preserves vision. This vegetable is also versatile, so you can add it to your meal in a variety of ways that cut across juices,

salads,   soups,   etc.

3. Almonds

Generally, nuts are tremendous, but almonds are excellent! Almonds are high in fiber, boost calcium absorption, and are a better snack alternative. You can get more protein from a quarter cup of almond than an egg, and they can be purchased easily from stores.

4. Tart Cherries

Tart cherries are used for baking, they come in frozen cans or as juices, but they are very healthy. Tart cherries contain anti-inflammatory nutrients that are great for managing pain. Tart cherries are flexible; they are a great addition to jam, smoothies, or mixed with other fruits.

5. Black beans

Black beans have a lot of omega-3 fats and cancer-fighting chemicals called flavonoids. If you can get canned beans, then high because they are very convenient but don't eat more than half a cup at once.

6. Blueberries

Berries are common in the U.S.A, and they contain Anthocyanidins, which gives the seed its peculiar color and health benefits. Blueberries are also rich in antioxidants; thus can lower the risk of diabetes and arthritis. Blueberries are also versatile as you can eat them all year round in varying dishes and multiple recipes.

7. Turmeric

In terms of spices, turmeric is an excellent addition to your meal. Turmeric contains curcumin, which teats infections. You can add turmeric to your soups and other snacks for vibrant color and flavor.

8. Sardines

Sardines taste like tuna and are a great way to get fish oil, vitamin D, and calcium. With sardines, you also get selenium, which is an antioxidant that keeps the immune system in great form to fight off cell damage. Always choose sardines without added salt for a healthy meal.

9. Beets

Beets are sweet, creamy, and great for women. Drinking a glass of beet juice (known as beetroot) can lower your blood pressure and reduce the risk of hypertension. The chemicals in the beet also combat inflammation, cancer, and heart disease.

10. Broccoli

Broccoli is an example of a cruciferous veggie just like cauliflower and Brussels Sprouts. One cup of Broccoli is enough to give your body its daily vitamin C requirement. Broccoli is green, can be eaten raw or slightly steamed, and is an excellent addition to any meal.

These foods are recommended for the prevention of illnesses and diseases in a woman's body. A lot of effort is required to stick to the right food routine long-term, but it is worth the effort. Your organization must be in great shape, and a combination of everything mentioned thus far with good food is ideal.

While focused on eating superfoods, you should also know the types of food to avoid. We live in a time with everything done swiftly, so now we've got fast cars, fats, emails, and even fast food (processed food). Such processed foods are problematic to the body, and they cause a lot of damage long-term.

Foods that contain excessive sugar are also a part of the problem; below, you will find a list of some of these foods. Please note that for some foods below, it is alright to have them occasionally, they become terrible for your health when you take them EXCESSIVELY!

With the list below, you will find healthy alternatives to the wrong foods.

List of foods to avoid

1. Ice cream

We all love ice-cream, but it contains sugar and is high in calories. With ice-cream, you can also overeat, which makes it a struggle for you.

The alternatives to ice-cream will be to settle for healthier brands that produce ice-cream with no sugar and fruits. You could also make homemade ice-cream using fruits.

2. Processed meat

People who eat a lot of processed meat have a higher chance of getting type 2 diabetes and heart disease.

Watch out for the source of your bacon, sausages, or pepperoni to ensure that there are no added artificial ingredients.

If you can avoid processed meat entirely, please do and if you can't buy from the local butcher.

3. Some fruit juice

Some fruit juices contain liquid sugar such that they may have more sugar than sodas like Coke. While some fruit juices have health benefits, you must read the labels to know the content and ascertain if it is healthy for you.

The alternative to store-bought and packaged fruit juice is freshly homemade juice without added sugars.

4. Candy bars

Candy bars are sweet but unhealthy because they are high in sugar, processed fats, and refined wheat flour. Another problem with the candy bar is that after consuming them, you will feel hungry for more, and this encourages a wrong eating circle.

Replace candy bars with fruit or dark chocolate.

5. Pastries, cookies, and cakes

Some pieces of bread, cake, and cookies are unhealthy when overeaten. The packaged cookies are made with more refined sugar and added fats, which are all wrong for the body. These are delicious treats, but they don't offer real nutrients to the body, and they are filled with preservatives.

If you can, please stay away from desserts. But if you cannot stay away then stick to Greek Yogurt, dark chocolates or fresh fruits (for example pineapple is excellent, and it's sweet).

6. French fries and potato chips

While white potatoes are healthy when boiled but French fries and potato chips are not. French fries and chips are high in calories, and they contain a high amount of acrylamides.

If you must consume potatoes, then it should be boiled and NOT fried! If you want that crunchy feel with what you eat, then eat nuts or baby carrots.

7. High-calorie coffee drink

Coffee is rich in antioxidants and offers a lot of benefits, but it becomes problematic when there are a lot of added syrups, sugars, and other additives. These additions are harmful to the body, and when a person takes on repeatedly in a day, it can cause harm to the body.

When you want to drink coffee, stick with plain coffee or add a small amount of heavy cream. You can also rely on full-fat milk as a great addition with little or no sugar.

8. Food with added sugar

You must limit or altogether avoid food with added sugar, artificial trans-fat, and refined sugar. Most of the foods on the shelves today are made with such ingredients, which is why you must read food labels before making a purchase.

The alternative is to go for nutrient-dense whole foods that include fresh fruits and veggies.

9. Most packaged and processed food

When grocery shopping, you will discover a lot of processed and packaged foods that are full of excess salt and sugar. Persistent intake of such foods is not suitable for your health, especially if you want to lose weight.

The alternative to such processed foods is whole and organic foods. Also, read food labels before buying them while adding more veggies to your diet.

10. Most pizzas

Pizza is trendy worldwide as the most preferred junk food, but most commercial pizzas made with unhealthy ingredients. Some of the elements include processed meat and refined dough with most pizzas high in calories.

You can get an alternative to pizza in some restaurants that contain healthy ingredients. Homemade pizza is also a more healthy choice if you use wholesome and organic ingredients.

The role that food plays in the health discourse is highly essential, and we must be mindful of what we eat. Now you know some of the superfoods to enjoy and the harmful foods to avoid, take action, and protect your body's system.

Aside from food, there is also a people angle to our story, and it begins with the next chapter. What kind of friends do you have around you? Who are the people that influence you? Are they positive or negative? Should you cut them off? Get answers and more in the next chapter.

Chapter Five
The people in your life

To be a healthy and wholesome woman, you must take a closer look at the people in your life and the role they play. We are made or broken by the relationships we tolerate in our lives, so don't undermine the value of people.

Women are surrounded by people from birth, girlfriends, boyfriends, exes, family members, etc. For some women, they don't have control over the people that come into their lives, and this is one way through which they end up with a lousy company.

Bad company is the company of those who are negative in their thinking. This company also includes those who do not motivate or inspire you and not add value to your life.

Relationships are a two-way street; others expect good vibes from us the same way we expect value and positive friendship. The first part of the narrative is for you to build yourself as a woman of importance so you can give what you expect.

You must understand that everyone carries energies within and around them. These energies are shared through relationships, and if you are spending time with a person that exhibits negative energy is unhealthy for you.

Some people drain you of your energy after spending time with them, while some others make you feel rejuvenated. That is the primary question you must ask when assessing your relationships, "How does this person make me feel?"

Don't get carried away by the moments you've had with the individual or the timeline you've known him/her. Some people don't let go of negative friends because they claim they've known them since childhood, which is not a good excuse.

Here is a scenario to bolster this idea:

Let us assume that there are two ladies named Lisa and Tracy. Lisa is a very optimistic individual who practices gratitude and is positive. Tracy, on the other hand, is quite pessimistic, brings down others to feel good, and is generally an angry person.

Lisa and Tracy became friends at work and started spending time with each other. While Lisa was helpful and friendly to others, Tracy was the opposite, this continued for a while with Lisa "Hoping" she can change her friend's character.

Without Lisa knowing it, she was subconsciously instilling some of Tracy's attributes. Soon enough, she started to see reasons to be mean to people and less of her positive self. Of course, Lisa's friends and family noticed the change, but she couldn't see it because she was influenced.

Now there are several real-life examples of Lisa and Tracy's situation, and if you look back at your life, you will agree that there are people who have been influential in your life. More importantly, there are also people you influence, which means that we have a responsibility to be great women as well.

If you are going to get the best out of life health-wise and live happily, you must be intentional about the people you allow into your circle or relationships. Relationships with the right people make life very fulfilling because the people we encounter can give us moments of lifetime happiness or pain.

Cutting people off

Many people are not aware of their ability to cut the wrong people off their lives. For such individuals, they become comfortable, get attached, and do not see the damage done to their lives by keeping the wrong company.

If you observe that a person makes you question your values or what you are capable of, then that person isn't right for you. If someone makes it easier for you to pretend to be what you are not, please note that it is time to cut him/her off.

You don't have to create a scene or quarrel to cut people off; you can gradually start by spending less time with that individual until there is no room for a connection anymore. If the person asks why you no longer spend time with them, let them know the reason and make it clear that if they don't intend changing, you wouldn't be close to them anymore.

Peace of mind is very crucial for the realization of excellent health in women. The wrong relationships can take away your order; as such, you have a responsibility to cut them off. Think about yourself like a well-watered garden with beautiful flowers that bloom and pretty butterflies around you.

Like every garden, weeds tend to show up. The plants in your garden refer to people that don't add value to your life in any way. Think about weeds and grass you see in a garden, what purpose do they serve? They do nothing disrupt, and a good gardener will take them out from the roots immediately.

If the gardener tolerates them, soon enough, the weeds will outgrow the flowers and take over the garden. The beauty of the garden will be lost, and it will take more time to restore the garden.

When you view your life as a precious garden, you will become mindful of the people you allow in and the people who influence your decisions. Some women drink alcohol excessively (irresponsible drinking behavior) because they are always with friends that do the same.

Influence is a potent tool that people can use against us, so please take charge of your life. Choose your friends wisely, and if your values do not align with that of a friend, cut the person off. This book is all about inspiring and motivating you to take action towards living a more meaningful life.

A fulfilling life is a healthy one, and the people in your life play a crucial role in helping you attain such fulfillment. You cannot accept people with uninspiring energies into your mental space, you are not Santa Clause, and it isn't your responsibility to make everyone happy.

Your happiness and satisfaction must come first and if someone or a group of persons threaten that, they've got to go. The women who enjoy health on all fronts are not always with the wrong crowd. If they find that they are with the wrong people, they cut off and create their circle by carefully choosing who will be in that circle.

Women need to inspire and uplift other women, so when you have friends that tear other women down soon enough, you will join them and do the same, when people show you who they believe them and decide if you want them in your life or not.

In some cases, people can change when they sense that you are making a withdrawal. But you must be mindful of such changes because they may be changing just to remain friends with you, which isn't good enough. If anyone wants to improve their personality, it should be because they recognize that there is a problem and sincerely want to fix it.

This chapter has been about the value of relationships and the role the connection with people play in your life. If you are with negative people, you will become negative; don't take this realization for granted!

As you cut off those wrong persons from your life, you will need to improve on your gratitude level. The next chapter will teach you all about being intentional with gratitude as you anticipate living a wholesome and purposeful life.

Chapter Six

The connection between gratitude and good health

When we talk about a complete, whole, and healthy woman, we are referring to a grateful lady who is thankful for life. Gratitude plays a role in helping you stay healthy, and if you didn't know this truth before now, it is not too late to start being thankful.

Yes, the world is full of challenges we deal with daily, from finances to being great moms, sisters, wives, friends, etc. Life doesn't give a breather hence the reason some persons resort to complaints and fail to see the good in their lives.

An ungrateful person is one who considers the challenges and problems of life and makes them focus daily. For such a woman, regardless of the heights, she attains in life, there will be reasons to complain. This chapter is telling you that a significant pathway to health is by maintaining an attitude of gratitude daily.

Ingratitude makes you vulnerable to worry, fear, anxiety, and other negative issues that affect your mental health. Also, being ungrateful for life has consequences for physical health; it may not be 100% visible, but it builds up gradually.

In some cases, women may not know that they're ungrateful people, so let us consider the signs of an ungrateful person.

Signs of an ungrateful person

- Consistent complaints about everything

- Never appreciative of spouse or kids

- Highlights the negative in every situation

- Lacks optimism

- Never content

- Always frowning thus leading to fast aging

- Quick to anger

- Being resentful of others

- A feeling of entitlement that demands from others without giving back

- Lack of patience

The signs above are a few of the symptoms of an ungrateful person, but from the short lost, you will agree that such people are all around us. It is okay to be realistic about issues, but you must avoid excessive focus on the negative side of things.

No one has a perfect life, and the grass is never greener on the other side. To be whole as a woman, you must be appreciative of your journey in life, be thankful for where you are now while anticipating where you want to be. Gratitude is the best make-up product you can use, it is free, and it cleanses you from the inside out.

When you are grateful, you open up your heart and life for positive experiences that bring so much joy. You will continuously be in a state of happiness, contentment with little or no worries about life. For you o fully understand this, you must get to know the benefits of gratitude.

The benefits of gratitude

Gratitude aids improved psychological health

Psychological health relates to how happy and content you are about life, are you satisfied within you? Do you smile to yourself or complain incessantly? For improved psychological health, you must be a person of gratitude, always look around you, and seek what to be thankful for that moment.

Things may not always go your way, but you have the power to make the most out of every situation. The situation will be exactly how you interpret it, be grateful for it, and it will be a positive experience!

With gratitude, you've got high self-esteem

Grateful people are known for their fantastic elf-esteem because they are comfortable in who they are, and they love themselves. Such persons have challenges, but their focus is on the good happening in their lives hence the reason they have such admirable self-esteem.

When a woman is confident, she will also be a great person in her relationships and her world generally. Never underestimate the value of gratitude, start today, and build it consistently.

Gratitude helps women sleep better

If you have been struggling with good sleep, it may be because you are worried, irritated, and ungrateful for what you do have. Don't consider what you don't have and focus on "being thankful for what is yours.

Women will sleep better, relax more, and be at ease with themselves when they always express gratitude. Good sleep leads to significant health experiences, which adds value to your life.

Gratitude improves physical health

Gratitude also improves your physical health because a grateful person is at peace, and she would have fewer reasons to fall ill. She wouldn't be stressed out, anxious, or depressed about life; in the last chapter, you will find the connection between ingratitude and illnesses.

If you want a wholesome health experience, start today by being a grateful person who is always thankful. Get rid of headaches and heartaches through intentional gratitude.

You will have productive relationships

Gratitude helps you build enriching relationships that stand the test of time. When you are a grateful person, you will be positively-oriented, which means that people will naturally gravitate towards you and want to be close to you.

Be known in your world as a person who comes alive with joy when you see others because you are grateful for them. This goal is achieved with consistent practice.

Now you know the signs of those who are not grateful and the importance of gratitude concerning your health and life. But there is a way to create an experience of appreciation and sustain it long-term. Below, you will find a section on how to build and maintain a life of gratitude.

How to build and maintain a life of gratitude

Say thank you every morning

Incorporating recognition into your morning routine is an excellent way of preserving gratitude long-term. In the morning, regardless of the tasks ahead and smile while welcoming the new day with thanks.

Don't wait for the annual thanksgiving season before expressing gratitude; it must begin with the smaller things. Wake up early in the morning, say thank you for being alive and for your incredible life. Before sleeping at night, say thank you for the remarkable day you had, all of these matters.

Celebrate those you love

The people you love are around you, and they help you establish balance with your relationships, are you grateful for them? Do you appreciate your partner, kids, employees, bosses, friends, and family?

An excellent way to show gratitude for them is by celebrating them whenever you can. By celebration, we don't mean breaking the bank but carrying out random acts of kindness to them. Give hugs, write spontaneous thank you notes and say the words "Thank you" to those you love.

Say thank you to those that render service

Another way to incorporate gratitude into your daily experience is by saying "Thank you" to those who provide services. For example, some people do not say thank you to the waiter or cab driver because they pay for the service.

Well, the fact that you pay for a service doesn't mean you shouldn't be thankful when it is rendered excellently. Practice this step every day, and you will realize that saying thank you will come naturally to you every time.

Find the good in every challenge

In every problem you encounter in life, please seek the silver lining as it will help you become grateful for the experience. A life of gratitude entails being thankful in good and bad times; this will help you remain positive all the time.

Being grateful amid trouble is a sign of strength, and it will lead you to live an enriching and healthy life.

Keep a gratitude journal

With a gratitude journal, you will be holding yourself accountable to the gratitude process and build consistency as well. Your journal can be a physical or online material where you write down details of the events you are most grateful for that day.

Spend time reading the journal regularly, and you will be reminded of the blessings and great things in your life. If you cannot write every day in your journal, don't beat yourself about it, be consistent.

A healthy life is a great one that requires a whole lot of commitment to many areas of our lives. One such area is the aspect of being grateful, and this chapter has shown you why and how you should be grateful.

Not every health challenge a woman deals with is caused by infections and diseases; sometimes, it relates to the things we do and the things we do not do to give us a fuller life. Remember always to say "Thank you" to the universe and those around you; it is a pathway to a healthier and wealthier life.

There is a spiritual connection we must consider in all of these. You will find a detailed analysis of that in the next chapter. Have you heard about the term "Chakra" before? Do you know that there are spiritual causes of diseases? Head over to the next section to discover more.

Chapter Seven

The Spiritual causes of diseases and the concept of chakras

We will round off this fantastic experience with a section on the spiritual aspect of being a healthy woman, which entails two significant theories. The first concept relates to the idea of the spiritual causes of diseases, while the second idea is all about chakras.

We will consider both ideas separately in subsections below, but they have a unified message. The message is that there is a spiritual notion of being a healthy woman, which is essential. Some women are not familiar with the spiritual narrative, while others who may be familiar with it don't know how to use it.

After this chapter, you will be more attuned to this spiritual side and become conscious of the vital role it plays in helping you become very healthy.

The Spiritual causes of diseases

Certain diseases have spiritual roots, and we will identify some of them in this section. But it doesn't end with identification as after identifying them, you will have to release yourself from the spiritual stronghold so you can be free.

Alzheimer's disease: Spiritually, this occurs by a refusal to deal with the world the way it is, hopelessness, and anger. When a person doesn't control her reaction to situations, she gets to deal with anger and despair.

Bladder problems: This problem happens when anxiety and the fear of letting go are present in a woman. Fear is a deal-breaker when it comes to mental health from the lenses of spirituality.

Cancer: The causes of this disease are traced to deep hurt, being hateful, and a longstanding resentment.

Diabetes: The spiritual cause of this disease is a longing for what might have been and a need to control it.

Endometriosis: the major causes are insecurity, frustration, and disappointment.

Fever: The spiritual cause of this health challenge is anger and burning up inside.

Glaucoma: When a person feels pressured from outstanding hurts, she will be overwhelmed by it, and it will lead to unforgiveness. All of these contribute to glaucoma.

Hepatitis: This disease caused by a resistance to change, anger, fear, and hatred.

Infection: Infections occur when a woman is irritated, annoyed, or angry.

Jaundice: Jaundice occurs when there is internal and external prejudice.

Kidney stones: This disease aggravates when a person has a lot of undissolved anger issues.

Lupus: the causes are anger, punishment (self-inflicted), and giving up easily.

Menstrual problems: this disease has a connection to fear of being unwanted, fear of aging, and self-rejection.

Nausea: The spiritual cause of vomiting is a rejection of an idea or experience.

Osteomyelitis: Anger, frustration, and a feel of being unsupported contribute to this disease.

Paralysis: this disease is caused by paralyzing thoughts and getting stuck.

Rash: The irritation you feel over delays and your immature way of getting attention are the causes of a rash on your skin.

Sores: caused by unexpressed anger that settles into your subconscious.

Tuberculosis: selfishness, possessiveness, and evil thoughts, especially towards revenge, are the causes of the disease.

Urinary infection: this infection occurs when a person is angry at the opposite sex, and when she blames others as well.

Vitiligo: the spiritual cause is when you don't feel like you belong to a group or when you think outside of things.

Warts: warts caused by frustration about the future, the belief in ugliness and anger.

We cannot highlight all the diseases with spiritual causes here, so the list above is in an alphabetical arrangement of at least one disease representing a letter. If you struggle with any of these diseases, reverse the causes and be at peace with yourself.

The concept of chakras

The term "Chakra" refers to a Sanskrit word that means wheel, which depicts an energy wheel that continuously rotates. Chakras are in the central spinal column and also located in the front and back parts of the body.

Seven important chakras vibrate at varying speed levels with the chakra at the root rotating at a slow speed while the one at the crown rotates at a higher rate. Every chakra has a complementary color with a single-use, and the rainbow inspires the colors.

But you may be wondering, how does the chakra story relate to good health?

Well, if the chakras are not balanced or if the energies are not connected, the life force of the person will become slow. The physical body will be easily susceptible to diseases, and it can affect the mind as well. The person with an unbalanced chakra will deal with a range of illnesses and other mental struggles that include negativity, doubt, fear, etc.

As such, a person having a balanced chakra is crucial for good health. The keyword here is "Balance" because there will be problems when the chakra is excessively open and when closed. Another question at this stage will be, "How can I balance my chakras?" To balance your chakras, you will need to work with crystals and gemstones.

Crystals and gemstones react to electricity that moves through the body if the energy is slow; the vibration from the stone will harmonize and stimulate it to strike a balance. To achieve this balance with gemstones, you must know the seven chakras and the right stone to use.

First Chakra

The first chakra is known as the root chakra located at the base of the spine, where it holds the needs for survival and safety. If this chakra is blocked, the woman will feel anxious, insecure, fearful, and other physical issues. The colors associated with this chakra include brown, black, and red, while the gemstones to use in achieving balance are black tourmaline, garnet, and smoky quartz.

Second Chakra

The second chakra is the sacred chakra, which is below the navel. This chakra holds the intuition, sexuality, and creativity of a person, and when balanced, the person feels free with others. When it is blocked, it will lead to physical problems that include constipation, muscle spasms, and large intestine. This chakra is orange, and the gemstones are carnelian agate, Tigers eye, and orange calcite.

Third Chakra

The solar plexus chakra is the third, located below the breastbone, and it is the center of passion, impulses, and strength. When the chakra is balanced, the person feels outgoing with a lot of self-respect and expressivity. When the chakra is blocked, the person will lack confidence and worry about what others think. The chakra is yellow, and the gemstones are Citrine, Topaz, and yellow calcite.

Fourth Chakra

This fourth chakra is the heart chakra at the breast bone, and it is the center of spirituality, compassion, and love. With this chakra, the person can give and receive love while connecting the body, mind, and spirit. When this chakra is blocked, the person struggles with heart attack, high blood pressure, and difficulty while breathing. The colors are green and pinks with Rose Quartz and watermelon tourmaline as the gemstones.

Fifth Chakra

The fifth chakra is a throat chakra located in the collarbone of the lower neck. This chakra is the center of communications and the expression of creativity while aiding speech. If the chakra is balanced, the individual will be inspired to be creative and artistically prompted. When the chakra is not stable, the person will be physically ill with ailments such as inflammation, back pain, and skin irritations. The color is light blue, and its gemstones include Azurite and Aquamarine.

Sixth Chakra

The sixth chakra is the third eye located above the physical eye, and it is the center of high intuition. With a balanced sixth chakra, the person will be attuned to her higher-self and purified from negative tendencies. When this chakra is unbalanced, she may experience eye strain, blurred vision, and headaches. The colors of this chakra are dark blue and purple with gemstones Amethyst, Lapis Lazuli, and Sodalite.

Seventh Chakra

The seventh chakra is the crown chakra behind the top of the skull and a center for enlightenment. A balanced seventh chakra means the ability to open up to the divine energy and gain access to the subconscious. If this chakra is unbalanced, the individual will experience depression and migraine headaches. The colors for this chakra are white and purple with Clear Quartz Crustal. Amethyst and Oregon Opail as the gemstones.

The use of chakras to strike a balance with the body's energies is an ancient revelation. With the help of a Chakra healing practitioner using the old skill, you can heal numerous diseases. Your body, emotions, mind, and spirit transforms through a balancing of the chakras.

Spirituality and health are two concepts that work together to achieve a goal with human well-being. When a person understands how to blend both ideas, she would also be able to live a full and productive life.

This last chapter has expressed the connection between health and spirituality, but it is up to you to use the information received. We will round up the journey, complete with a concluding section that urges you to take action NOW.

Conclusion

When we started on this journey, we mentioned a statement of the fact that women are special, and you just proved how special you are by reading through from the beginning of this book to this point. You deserve a pat and a great lady high-five, well done!

However, reading isn't enough, and finishing this book isn't the end of the journey. On the contrary, now that you have finished reading, your journey of implementation just started. There is a disturbing trend with most readers, especially in this social media age; some readers learn a lot with zero application.

You cannot be a healthy woman based on what you read; you can only be that kind of woman based on what you execute. No one cares about what you know; they only care about what you DO. It is possible to know all the details in this book and more without making significant progress in your life, but this shouldn't be the goal.

The goal for every woman should be top read, discover, learn, and then implement. Execution completes the learning circle, and we are using this concluding section to drive the point home.

At this stage, you need to ask a vital question, "What am I going to do with everything I've learned?" You need to translate knowledge gained into real-life experiences by acting on the information.

The chapters above cut across numerous aspects of your life, which means you can start implementing the ideas one after the other. Don't wait until it "feels" right or when something serious happens to you before taking a step. The best time to bring the words to life is now, and it must be consistently implemented for you to get the value of the experience.

There are so many books out there on women's health and other genres, so it is safe to say we don't have an information problem in the world. If we don't lack information, how come women are still mostly unhealthy? The answer to the question is the fact that while we don't have an information problem, we do have an implementation challenge.

People love to read, but not many act on what they read. This concluding section is a timely reminder to you that knowledge only makes sense when a person acts on it. Don't put this book down until you have curated an execution plan. Go back to some of the chapters and sections to reread them until you get an idea of how you are going to implement the suggestions.

Yes, you are born unique, but you've got to bring that inner sparkle to life through deliberate action backed by impactful information. Of course, you are not expected to act on everything immediately because it's a lot across varying aspects.

What you can do is to start with the part that is most important to you, perfect it and then move on to the next one. If you can continue with this pattern, you will surely get the value of the book now and in the future. You've got to be very passionate about an idea for you to succeed while executing it, build passion and resilience will become natural to you.

There is much to achieve when you are in the right place, so please take execution seriously from this point. You will surely enjoy the implementation process as you add value to your life through action.

Remain a wholesome and healthy woman!

Best wishes.

www.ingramcontent.com/pod-product-compliance
Lightning Source LLC
Chambersburg PA
CBHW031135250726
48655CB00002B/689